The Ageless
Vitality
A Holistic Approach to Wellness and Longevity

IOANA LEE

Written by: Ioana Lee

Printed by: (optional)

Printed in the United States of America
Printing Year, 2023
ISBN 0-0000000-0-0

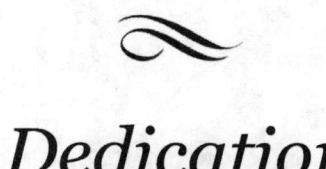

Dedication

Table of Contents

About The Author

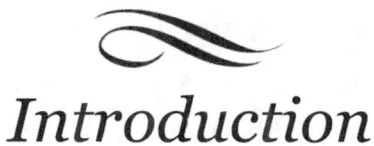

Introduction

It's not unusual for us to find ourselves reflecting on the true meaning of aging and wellbeing in a culture that seems to be perpetually on the hunt for the fountain of youth. We experience many turning points and obstacles as we move through life, and it is at these times that we truly understand the importance of preserving our health. When I think back on my own experience navigating the complexities of aging, I realize how crucial it is to have a holistic approach that takes into account one's physical, mental, and emotional health. I am quite excited to share this book with you, "The Ageless Vitality: A Holistic Approach to Wellness and Longevity," which aims to empower and encourage readers to enjoy a vibrant and meaningful existence.

Objectives of the book

This book's main goals are to demystify the idea of aging and offer insightful information on the complex realm of wellness. We will go on a voyage of self-discovery and arm ourselves with the knowledge necessary to manage the aging process with grace and energy by examining the subjects of diet, physical activity, mental well-being, and social connections. We will learn the secrets of sustaining a vigorous and satisfying life as we age through personal experiences, scientific research, and useful advice.

Overview of following chapters

Let's now take a quick look at the chapters that are still to come, each one packed with knowledge and direction to help us better comprehend wellness and aging.

By examining the fundamentals of wellbeing and the aging process, Chapter II will establish the groundwork. We will learn more about the complex systems at work by exploring the biology and psychological aspects of aging. We will learn the significance of adopting a holistic strategy for aging in this chapter, one that takes into account every aspect of our wellbeing.

The fundamental building blocks of nutrition and hydration will be revealed in Chapter III. We'll delve into the significance of a balanced diet and examine the crucial elements our bodies need to function properly. We will also explore how important hydration is for enhancing general health and reversing the effects of aging.

We will explore the world of superfoods and anti-aging in Chapter IV. We shall discover a wide variety of superfoods and their special benefits by comprehending the power of antioxidants and their function in the aging process. The immense potential that resides within the field of nutrition will be made clear to us in this chapter.

The realm of supplements will be introduced to in Chapter V, along with its significance as we become older. We will examine nutritional supplements that are crucial for our health, including vitamins, minerals, probiotics, omega-3 fatty acids, and collagen. We will learn how to navigate the supplement industry and make wise decisions by balancing the advantages and disadvantages.

In Chapter VI, we examine the definition and significance of the clean living lifestyle. We'll learn about doable strategies for integrating clean living into our daily lives, from utilizing non-toxic household products to selecting natural and organic meals. We will also examine how minimizing plastic use improves the environment and learn how a healthy lifestyle slows down aging.

The transforming impact of physical activity on our wellbeing will be highlighted in Chapter VII. We will find the solution to achieving our maximum potential as we age by learning about the advantages of regular exercise and investigating several types of exercise, such as aerobic workouts, strength training, yoga, and Pilates. This chapter will also offer doable recommendations for working exercise into our daily schedules.

In Chapter VIII, the crucial link between mental health and aging will take center stage. We will look into the practices and methods that support mental health, such as stress reduction, mindfulness, meditation, and cognitive training. We may harness the enormous power of mental health and its profound effects on the aging process by cultivating a happy outlook.

We shall examine the frequently underrated role that sleep plays in both our general health and the aging process in Chapter IX. We will explore how to enhance the quality of our sleep as well as the role that sleep plays in renewing our bodies and minds. We can move toward a more energetic and young existence by addressing typical sleep problems.

The significant influence that social relationships have on our wellbeing will be discussed in Chapter X. We will learn techniques to develop and sustain healthy relationships through an investigation of the complex relationship between social engagement and aging. This chapter will also demonstrate the joy and life-changing potential of community involvement.

We'll wrap up our voyage in Chapter XI by summarizing the major themes covered in the book. With the information and inspiration gleaned from these pages, we will urge readers to set out on their own individual journey toward holistic well-being. We'll share our final insights and motivations as we say goodbye, encouraging each reader to follow their own particular route to a rich and satisfying life.

Let's embrace the knowledge found in these pages as we set out on this educational adventure together and use it to empower ourselves to live vibrant, meaningful, and joyful lives. The possibilities are unlimited as the adventure waits. Let's explore the core concepts of wellness and aging to learn the real keys to a life well-lived.

1. Understanding Wellness and Aging

We're glad you're here as we continue our exploration of wellness and aging. We will delve into the fundamental nature of wellness and examine its profound relationship to the aging process in this chapter. It's imperative that we first comprehend what wellbeing really entails before we start our investigation.

Wellness is a holistic state of well-being that includes physical, mental, and emotional health; it goes much beyond simply being free from disease. It is a dynamic and always changing idea that entails nurturing and balancing every element of our lives in order to feel fulfillment and harmony. In addition to our physical bodies, our brains, emotions, relationships, and even our connection to the outside world are all included in our definition of wellness. Our experience of aging and the caliber of our lives are shaped by the complex interplay of all these factors.

Having a good understanding of aging

As we carry on with our investigation, we must face the irrefutable truth of aging. The consequences of aging can be seen in both our bodies and thoughts, and it is a normal and unavoidable component of the human experience. Let's look at the aging process from both a biological and psychological angle to acquire a deeper understanding.

A Biological Point of View

In terms of biology, aging is a result of a complex interplay of genetic, environmental, and lifestyle factors that over time influence how our cells, tissues, and organs operate. Our bodies undergo cellular changes with time, including a fall in cellular repair systems and a reduction in the creation of crucial chemicals. Numerous age-related illnesses and diseases can develop as a result of these changes. However, it's crucial to remember that while aging is a natural process, there are a number of lifestyle decisions we can make to affect the speed at which it happens and how it affects our health.

From a psychological point of view

Beyond its physical effects, aging has a significant psychological effect on people. The emotional and cognitive changes that take place as we get older are covered by the psychological perspective on aging. It comprises dealing with the difficulties and rewards of aging, finding meaning and purpose in later life, and adjusting to new life circumstances. For the purpose of promoting mental health and ensuring a positive attitude on life as we age, it is essential to understand the psychological components of aging.

The significance of a comprehensive approach to aging

We can now see the innate relationship between wellbeing and the aging process after exploring their definitions. Physical, mental, and emotional aspects of aging are all present, and it would be insufficient to focus solely on one of these aspects. This insight emphasizes the significance of taking an all-encompassing approach to aging.

A holistic view of aging recognizes the numerous connections between our health and other facets of our existence. It acknowledges the necessity of providing our bodies with the right nourishment, frequent exercise, care for our mental and emotional health, and the development of deep social ties. We can improve our quality of life, improve our well-being, and age with grace and vigor by adopting a holistic approach.

We shall delve further into the various facets of wellness and aging in the sections that follow in this chapter. We'll go over the relevance of eating right and being hydrated, the function of superfoods and supplements, the connection between exercise and mental health, the value of getting enough sleep, the value of social connections, and much more. We can start a revolutionary journey toward holistic well-being and graceful aging by arming ourselves with knowledge and wisdom.

So let's get off on this illuminating journey together as we learn how to embrace wellness and aging. Get ready to explore your own potential and the transformational power of nurturing your mind, body, and spirit. The road to a healthy and happy old age is here!

Defining wellness

The term "wellness" has become increasingly prevalent in today's culture, usually referring to a condition of complete physical and mental health. But what does it mean to be healthy, exactly? We need to delve further into the many facets of wellbeing if we are to grasp it properly.

Wellness, in its essence, is more than just the absence of sickness. It entails thriving in all aspect of one's life, physically, mentally, and socially. It's the science and practice of making sure we have all we need to grow and develop in every area of our life.

Physical Wellness

When we say we are physically well, we mean that our bodies and daily routines are healthy and effective. It entails making changes to one's lifestyle that enhance health and vitality, such as increasing physical activity, eating a balanced diet, getting enough sleep, and dealing effectively with stress. The pursuit of physical wellbeing involves being attuned to one's physical demands and taking preventative measures to ensure and improve health.

Mental Wellness

When our minds are strong and clear, we are mentally well. It includes our intelligence, emotional stability, and general psychological health. Positive thinking, efficient stress management, the development of coping mechanisms, and participation in mentally stimulating activities are all necessary for achieving mental wellbeing. Self-awareness, mindfulness, reaching out for help when you need it, and a balanced existence are all part of this.

Emotional Wellness

When we are able to recognize, name, and control our feelings, we are said to be emotionally well. Understanding oneself, learning to manage one's emotions, and forming supportive bonds are all part of this. Activities that enhance emotional well-being, such as hobbies, self-care, and reaching out for emotional assistance when needed, are advocated for under the concept of emotional wellbeing.

Social Wellness

Connections and interactions with other people are at the heart of what it means to be socially healthy. It involves establishing and maintaining strong connections with others, feeling like we belong in our communities, and making meaningful contributions to those places. Open dialogue, compassion, and caring for one another are hallmarks of a healthy social life. Fostering friendships, going out, volunteering, and accepting others' differences are all part of this.

Spiritual Wellness

The pursuit of a higher meaning and purpose in life is at the heart of spiritual well-being. It entails getting in touch with our inner selves, discovering our core beliefs, and figuring out what gives our lives meaning. Meditation, introspection, doing work that reflects our values, spending time in nature, or communicating with a higher power are all ways to improve our spiritual health, but there are many other ways as well.

Environmental Wellness

The concept of environmental wellbeing highlights the relationship between human health and the state of the natural world. It entails learning how our actions affect the earth and then choosing actions that are good for long-term sustainability and ecological harmony. Living in tune with nature, recycling, conserving resources, and backing environmental protection efforts are all aspects of environmental wellbeing.

All of these aspects of health have an effect on one another. Real health is the result of paying attention to and caring for all aspects of one's being in order to develop a life that is both balanced and fulfilling. Discovering oneself, caring for oneself, and bettering oneself is an endless process.

By committing to the idea of wellbeing, we can work toward a life that is robust, meaningful, and joyful. It gives us the ability to determine our own fate and make deliberate decisions that improve our health and happiness. So, let's start this road of self-improvement by acknowledging the many facets of health and the power we have to create a life we love.

Understanding the aging process

The natural and intricate process of aging is something we all must face as we travel through life. Changes in our bodies and minds as we age affect how we see the world and how we interact with others. It is essential to look at aging from both a biological and psychological standpoint if we are to have a whole picture of it.

Biological perspective

Aging is a complex biological process that is affected by a wide range of variables, such as one's genes, one's lifestyle, and one's surroundings. A decrease in the body's capacity to repair and regenerate cells, tissues, and organs is one of the hallmarks of aging at the cellular level. The decline in vital biological systems causes age-related changes in appearance and makes us more susceptible to age-related disorders.

Telomeres, the protective caps at the ends of chromosomes, shorten as a result of the biological aging process. With each cell division, telomeres gradually shorten until they reach a critical length, at which point the cell enters a senescent state or dies. Telomere shortening is thought to play a role in the aging process as a whole.

And oxidative stress is a major contributor to the aging process. The free radicals produced by environmental stressors like pollution and UV radiation can harm cells and DNA throughout a person's lifetime. Damage from oxidative stress can accumulate over time, reducing cell function and speeding up the aging process. Certain nutrients and the body's own production of antioxidants are useful in combating free radicals and oxidative stress.

Hormone levels also fluctuate naturally as people age. Menopause is an example of a natural drop in reproductive hormone production that causes a number of changes in a woman's body and hormone levels. As men age, their testosterone levels naturally decrease, which has negative effects on their vitality, muscle mass, and libido.

Psychological perspective

The psychological aspects of aging have an impact on our mental, emotional, and social health. Brain function, memory, and processing speed all decline with age. Aging is associated with a natural drop in cognitive capacities, yet this decline need not be catastrophic. Supporting cognitive health and slowing age-related cognitive decline can be achieved through engaging in mentally stimulating activities, maintaining social relationships, and adopting a healthy lifestyle.

The emotional experiences we have as we age can vary widely. Some people may experience happiness and fulfillment in old age, while others may struggle with grief, loneliness, and nervousness. Changes in circumstances, such as retirement or the death of a loved one, can have an effect on one's mental and emotional health. To overcome these emotional obstacles and keep one's mental health intact, one must practice resilience, adopt a positive outlook, and surround oneself with supportive people.

The psychological effects of aging are also heavily influenced by social variables. Maintaining one's mental and emotional health requires having strong social ties and a feeling of belonging to a group. An increased risk of physical and mental health problems has been related to loneliness and social isolation, which can be more common among the elderly. Purpose, fulfillment, and psychological health can all be enhanced via the cultivation and maintenance of social relationships, engagement in community activities, and building bridges across generations.

Moreover, one's own mental reaction to aging might be affected by one's own attitudes and thoughts regarding the process. Self-esteem, resilience, and quality of life can all benefit from adopting a positive outlook and rejecting ageist prejudices.

Importance of a holistic approach to aging

The development of successful techniques to promote healthy aging requires an appreciation for the multifaceted character of the aging process. Aging is a complex combination of biological and psychological processes, as well as social and environmental contexts. Therefore, it is crucial to take a holistic view of aging if one is to achieve optimum health and quality of life.

Health on all levels—physical, mental, and social—are acknowledged to be interdependent and mutually important in a holistic perspective. When people take care of their mental, physical, and spiritual health all at once, they are better able to meet the changing demands of aging.

Supporting the body's resilience and reducing age-related health disorders can be accomplished by regular exercise, a balanced diet, and sufficient sleep. Enhancing one's mental and emotional health through mentally challenging pursuits, mindful awareness, and the pursuit of new experiences. A sense of purpose, belonging, and fulfillment can be cultivated by the nurturing of social ties, the active pursuit of community engagement, and the maintenance of a positive outlook.

Preventative care and early intervention are valued by those who have a holistic view of aging. By making healthy decisions and getting frequent checkups, people can identify and manage health issues early, improving their quality of life and boosting their chances of gracefully aging.

Taking a comprehensive view of aging requires knowledge of the biological and psychological aspects of the aging process. One's quality of life in old age can be improved by cultivating tactics that enhance one's physical health, cognitive function, and relationships with others. The process of getting older is reframed as something positive: a chance to gain experience and insight while continuing on the path to complete well-being.

Importance of a holistic approach to aging

It is becoming increasingly apparent that a holistic approach is necessary for fostering general well-being and maximizing the quality of our lives as we travel the path of aging. This all-encompassing viewpoint acknowledges that there is more to aging than just our bodies. It recognizes the complex relationship between one's physical, mental, and social well and stresses the significance of fostering all three. Let's have a look at the reasons why a comprehensive perspective on aging is so crucial.

Enhancing overall well-being

The effects of aging are felt across our entire existence, not just our bodies as they weaken over time. The best way to improve our health as a whole is to work on it from every angle at once. Taking a more all-encompassing view of our well-being helps us age more gracefully because it fosters a state of equilibrium and harmony. Taking care of our bodies, minds, hearts, and souls by eating right, exercising regularly, getting plenty of sleep, and maintaining positive relationships lays the groundwork for a rich and full life.

Preventing and managing age-related conditions

Taking a more all-encompassing view of the aging process allows us to proactively prevent age-related illnesses and better manage ongoing health issues. Chronic diseases including cardiovascular disease, diabetes, and some forms of cancer can be avoided through emphasizing regular physical activity, embracing a nutrient-rich diet, and engaging in self-care activities. The risk of cognitive decline and mental health disorders may also be reduced if we attend to the psychological aspects of aging, such as stress management and building resilience.

Promoting cognitive health

Taking a comprehensive approach can help prevent cognitive loss, which is commonly associated with aging. Reading, puzzles, and learning new skills are all great ways to keep the mind sharp and stave off the effects of aging on the brain. Engaging in mentally taxing activities like group talks or educational programs, and keeping up with one's social circle, both contribute to a healthy mind. We can maintain our mental acuity and improve our brain health in general by adopting a more balanced diet and lifestyle.

Fostering emotional resilience

Maintaining your mental health is essential for growing older gracefully. We may build emotional resilience and deal with the difficulties of aging by taking care of our mental and emotional health through approaches like mindfulness, self-reflection, and stress management. When we take a more holistic view, we are more likely to allow ourselves to feel our feelings, reach out for help when we need it, and develop an optimistic outlook. If we take care of our mental health, we'll be better prepared to handle the inevitable emotional ups and downs that come with becoming older.

Cultivating meaningful social connections

Maintaining meaningful relationships is essential to our health at every stage of life, but especially as we get older. In order to age healthily, it's important to cultivate and sustain meaningful relationships with others. Combating social isolation, enhancing our sense of belonging, and contributing to overall happiness and life satisfaction can be achieved through regular social interactions, participation in community activities, and cultivation of a support network. Having strong friendships can help you feel less lonely, protect you from developing mental health problems, and boost your happiness.

Embracing the wisdom of aging

Finally, a comprehensive view of aging enables us to value the insights and perspective that come with greater years lived. It inspires us to take stock of our experiences, appreciate our virtues, and rejoice in our successes. By appreciating the insights that come from years of experience, we can develop a more optimistic view of aging, one that welcomes the chances it presents for personal development, social impact, and legacy building.

Promoting general health, preventing age-related diseases, nurturing cognitive health, building emotional resilience, making and maintaining meaningful social connections, and accepting the knowledge that comes with aging all require a comprehensive perspective on aging. To age with elegance and vitality, we must take into account the interdependence of our physical, mental, and social selves on a journey toward holistic aging. Let us embrace this holistic method, for it is the key to a rich and rewarding old age.

2. *The Basics of Nutrition and Hydration*

In this chapter, we will set out on a quest to learn why proper nutrition and hydration are so crucial to our well-being and longevity. As we examine the significant effect that food and water have on our health, the old adage "you are what you eat" rings truer than ever.

Human health is predicated on the fuel we provide our bodies, which is the food we eat. Maintaining health, energy, and lifespan through diet is the foundation. It's not enough to just watch our caloric intake or adhere to the latest diet fad; we also need to ensure that our bodies are receiving the nutrients they require. A healthy, well-rounded diet is a powerful tool for maintaining health and vitality into old life.

Examining the nutrients our bodies need to function at peak levels is crucial to grasping the importance of a well-rounded diet. Vitamins, minerals, carbs, proteins, fats, and fiber all play important roles in keeping us alive and allowing our bodies to function normally. Each vitamin contributes in its own way to our health and wellness, therefore it's important to get enough of them all.

Vitamins and minerals, sometimes known as micronutrients, play an important role in a number of essential biological processes. They help keep our immune system healthy, contribute to cellular repair and growth, and aid in the creation of energy. The vast potential for improving our health that may be unlocked by learning about the function of these micronutrients and including them in our diets is only waiting to be tapped.

In addition to fueling and repairing our bodies, macronutrients like carbs, proteins, and fats are essential. Our cells require carbohydrates for energy, proteins for repair and growth, and lipids for hormone production and thermal regulation. The key to meeting the needs of the body and being healthy is adopting a well-rounded perspective on these macronutrients.

Fiber's importance in maintaining a healthy weight, controlling blood sugar, and promoting digestive health is sometimes understated. It helps break down food, keeps you from being constipated, and even benefits your heart. Fiber-rich meals are beneficial to our health because they aid in the proper functioning of our digestive systems.

While discussing the significance of nutrition, it is imperative to also highlight the significance of water intake. The human body relies on water, the "elixir of life," to function properly and stay healthy. Adequate hydration is essential for the proper functioning of every cell, tissue, and organ in the human body.

As a means of conveyance, water brings oxygen and nutrients to our cells and takes away toxins. It helps break down food, keeps the temperature steady, cushions the internal organs, and keeps the joints lubricated. The skin, the brain, and the body all benefit from being well hydrated.

The importance of being well hydrated increases with aging. Dehydration is more common in the elderly because their sensation of thirst may be diminished. Fatigue, dizziness, constipation, and even memory loss are just some of the symptoms of dehydration. By giving water its due, we can help our bodies continue working at peak efficiency and encourage proper maturation.

In this chapter, we'll take a closer look at the components of a healthy diet and the importance of striking a balance between them. We'll learn why certain nutrients are so crucial, and we'll explore the many tasty and healthy food options that exist. In addition, we will discuss the value of water, dispel myths, and offer suggestions for fulfilling the body's water requirements.

Get ready to learn about the best ways to fuel your body and support your health as you age by going on a journey of nourishment and hydration. Discovering the transformational power of a healthy food and sufficient water intake together is the key to a life of vitality and flourishing health.

The importance of a balanced diet

In today's fast-paced, convenience-focused society, it's easy to lose sight of the importance of eating a variety of nutritious foods every day. What we put into our body, however, has a significant effect on our health, happiness, and the rate at which we age. A well-rounded diet is the cornerstone of good health, as it supplies the majority of the nutrients our systems require. Discussing why a healthy diet is so crucial.

Nourishing our bodies

Fundamentally, a healthy diet is one that nourishes our bodies by providing the essential nutrients needed for optimal performance. It gives our cells what they need to function, helps them grow and mend, and allows our internal systems to do their complicated jobs. In addition to helping our immune systems function properly, minerals and vitamins also promote strong bones and organs. Adopting a healthy, well-rounded diet gives us the energy to blossom.

Disease prevention

A healthy diet is an important tool in the fight against illness. Heart disease, diabetes, and some forms of cancer are only some of the chronic illnesses that have been linked to dietary patterns. Fruits, vegetables, whole grains, lean meats, and healthy fats are just some examples of nutrient-dense foods. These foods provide us with the antioxidants, vitamins, minerals, and phytochemicals that strengthen our immune systems and protect our cells from free radical damage. A healthy diet can protect us from dangerous illnesses by providing our bodies with the nutrients they need to function at their best.

Weight management

A balanced diet is crucial to obtaining and maintaining a healthy weight, which is vital for optimal health. Eating a balanced diet that includes a wide variety of foods in reasonable serving sizes will help us prevent overeating while yet meeting our nutritional needs. A healthy diet contains a variety of nutrients that boost our metabolism and aid in fat loss, and it also helps us feel full longer, reducing the likelihood that we will overeat. It gives us the tools to get in tune with our bodies, which is crucial for developing a positive perspective toward food and achieving sustainable weight loss.

Energy and vitality

Our health and vigor are directly affected by the things we eat. A healthy diet provides the right mix of carbs, proteins, and fats to fuel our cells and keep us going throughout the day. It ensures mental clarity and attention by providing the building blocks for a healthy brain. To thrive and participate completely in our daily lives, we need to provide our bodies with the high-quality nutrition they need to function optimally.

Gut health and digestion

A healthy diet is essential for good digestion and the maintenance of a healthy digestive tract. The gut microbiome benefits from a varied and fiber-rich diet by encouraging the growth of good bacteria there. This, in turn, improves digestion, strengthens the immune system, and increases nutritional absorption. By prioritizing a diet that's both nutritious and varied, you may improve your gut health and your overall health.

Mental well-being

A well-rounded diet not only improves our physical health, but also our state of mind. Nutrients like omega-3 fatty acids, B vitamins, and antioxidants have been linked to improved brain function and emotional stability. A diet rich in these nutrients has been shown to improve mental clarity, stabilize mood, and lower the chance of developing mental health conditions. Emotional and mental toughness can be enhanced through eating a healthy, well-rounded diet.

Keeping our diets well-rounded is crucial to our health, happiness, and longevity. It nourishes our minds and bodies by giving us the fuel we need to do our daily activities and by helping us maintain a healthy weight. A healthy lifestyle, including eating a well-rounded diet, gives us the tools we need to age gracefully and fully enjoy life to the fullest.

Essential nutrients for the body

To properly nourish our bodies and achieve peak health, knowledge of the significance of important nutrients is crucial. These nutrients are the backbone of our bodies, essential to our survival, health, and even the aging process itself. Let's take a closer look at the vital nutrients our bodies require and the crucial functions they play in ensuring we stay healthy.

Vitamins

Vitamins are chemical substances that play important roles in maintaining good health. They are essential for normal metabolic processes, immune system functioning, cell division, and development. Vitamin C and the B vitamins are examples of water-soluble vitamins, while vitamins A, D, E, and K are examples of fat-soluble vitamins. Each vitamin has a unique purpose and can be found only in certain foods. Vitamin D, which helps the body absorb calcium, may be created when exposed to sunshine, while vitamin C, which is found in citrus foods and leafy greens, boosts immunological function.

Minerals

Minerals are inorganic compounds required for many physiological processes. They're essential for skeletal health, fluid homeostasis, nerve conduction, and energy generation. Calcium, iron, potassium, magnesium, and zinc are just a few examples of crucial minerals. Dairy products and dark green vegetables are excellent sources of calcium, whereas lean meats, legumes, and fortified cereals are good sources of iron.

Carbohydrates

The majority of the energy that the body uses comes from carbohydrates. They're essential for keeping you energized throughout the day, from working out to keeping your mind sharp. Sugars found in fruits and sweets are examples of simple carbs, while complex carbohydrates include things like whole grains, legumes, and vegetables. Because of their higher fiber content and slower digestion, complex carbohydrates are preferable for providing constant energy throughout the day.

Proteins

Proteins have crucial roles in cell division, wound healing, and tissue preservation. Amino acids are the building blocks for all the different proteins in the body. Proteins are required for cellular processes like muscular growth, immunological response, and enzyme synthesis. Lean meats, chicken, fish, dairy products, legumes, and nuts are all excellent protein sources.

Fats

Fats, despite their bad rap, have their place in a healthy diet. They're important for producing hormones, absorbing nutrients, and shielding inside organs, and they also provide a concentrated source of energy. Avocados, almonds, and olive oil are all good sources of healthy unsaturated fats, but fried foods and processed snacks are high in unhealthy saturated and trans fats.

Fiber

The body cannot break down fiber, hence it is considered a "good carb." It plays a crucial role in preserving good digestion, controlling blood sugar, and making you feel full. Fruits, vegetables, whole grains, legumes, and nuts are all good sources of fiber.

There is a specific function served by each of these vital nutrients in maintaining good health. They complement one another, therefore eating a wide variety of nutrient-dense foods is important for getting enough of them in your diet.

Fruits, vegetables, whole grains, lean proteins, and healthy fats supply the nutrition our bodies need to flourish, and hence promote good aging. We can better fuel our bodies and achieve our full potential if we have a firm grasp on the function of these vital nutrients. Prioritizing the consumption of these critical nutrients, which provide us with the basis for vigorous and meaningful lives, becomes increasingly important as we age.

The role of hydration in overall health and aging

In addition to being essential to overall health, being hydrated can slow down the aging process. In order to carry out a vast array of physiological processes, our systems are completely reliant on water. In this article, we will discuss the importance of staying hydrated and how it can affect your health as you age.

Proper bodily function

Everything in our bodies, from cells to tissues to organs, is mostly water. It plays a vital role in chemical processes, nutrient absorption, and waste removal. The cardiovascular system, the digestive system, and the body's ability to regulate its temperature all benefit from being well hydrated. It aids in healthy blood volume maintenance, facilitates effective digestion, and contributes to efficient temperature regulation.

Nutrient transport and waste removal

The distribution of nutrients throughout the body relies heavily on water. It aids in the transportation of nutrients to our cells, increasing the likelihood that those nutrients will be taken in and used. Water also aids in the elimination of waste and pollutants via perspiration, urination, and defecation. The body's ability to carry nutrients and eliminate waste products is directly related to how well hydrated it is.

Joint and muscle health

Joint and muscle health depend on enough hydration. Water acts as a lubricant, reducing friction between the body's moving parts and reducing the risk of injury. It aids in the delivery of nutrients that promote joint health to the cartilage. Muscle function is improved, and cramps and exhaustion are avoided, when you drink enough water before, during, and after your workout. Keeping yourself hydrated helps maintain your body's mobility, strength, and performance.

Skin health and anti-aging

Skin health and the appearance of youthfulness depend critically on proper hydration. Hydrating with water helps the skin retain its natural suppleness and smooth out fine lines and wrinkles. It aids in the transport of vital nutrients to skin cells, which in turn helps the skin glow. In addition, flushing out impurities through perspiration helps maintain a healthy glow and clear skin. Maintaining an adequate water intake helps maintain the health and beauty of the skin from the inside out.

Cognitive function and mental well-being

The effects of dehydration on one's ability to think and feel good are substantial. The effects of dehydration on cognition, attention, and mood have been well-documented. A well-hydrated brain is one that can think clearly, focus intently, and remember details. Maintaining an adequate water intake has been linked to improved cognitive performance, a more buoyant disposition, and a decreased risk of cognitive deterioration.

Energy and fatigue prevention

Water is crucial for avoiding weariness and keeping up one's energy levels. Fatigue, drowsiness, and a general lack of energy are among symptoms of dehydration, which can also impair one's ability to think and function. By taking in plenty of fluids, we supply our bodies with the hydration they need to create the energy that powers our muscles and brains. The key to keeping our youthful vitality as we age is drinking enough water.

Hydration takes on an even greater significance as we get older. Dehydration is more common in the elderly because their sensation of thirst may be diminished. Constipation, urinary tract infections, and an increased risk of falls are just some of the health problems that can result from being chronically dehydrated. Conditions associated with aging, such as joint discomfort and cognitive decline, might be made worse by this. Therefore, it is especially important for senior citizens to pay close attention to their hydration levels and make sure they drink enough water throughout the day.

In order to keep in good health and age gracefully, it's crucial to drink plenty of water. The body's systems, including the joints, muscles, skin, brain, and digestive tract, all benefit from a constant supply of hydrating fluids. Let's make water consumption a top priority, because it's good for our health, our bodies, and the quality of our lives as we age.

3. Superfoods and Anti-*Aging*

In this chapter, we'll delve into the definition of "superfoods," learn how antioxidants help prevent aging, and identify a wide variety of foods that pack a nutritional punch. Get ready to go out on a quest to learn how superfoods can be used to promote healthy and youthful aging.

The term "superfood" is used to describe a distinct group of foods that are extremely high in beneficial nutrients. They include several health-promoting nutrients such vitamins, minerals, antioxidants, and other bioactive substances. Superfoods are very beneficial since they not only nourish the body but also have qualities that help prevent chronic diseases, strengthen the immune system, and make us seem younger.

Understanding the function of antioxidants in the aging process is crucial to appreciating the value of superfoods. Antioxidants are substances that aid in the neutralization of free radicals, which are produced as byproducts of normal body activities and can lead to oxidative stress if not dealt with. Damage to our cells and DNA caused by oxidative stress contributes to premature aging and an upped chance of developing chronic diseases.

Antioxidants are essential for preventing the harm caused by oxidative stress. Antioxidants help prevent cell damage, promote organ and tissue health, and keep us feeling young and energized by scavenging free radicals. Antioxidant-rich foods, such as superfoods, have been shown to slow down the aging process, improve cellular health, and boost well-being.

Let's explore the fascinating realm of superfoods and learn about all the wonderful advantages they provide. The wonderful range of superfoods available to us includes, but is not limited to, berries, leafy greens, nuts and seeds, fatty fish, turmeric, green tea, and dark chocolate. The tremendous potential of these nutrient-dense foods for fostering robust health, fortifying resistance to aging, and cultivating overall well-being can be accessed through regular consumption.

In the following sections of this chapter, we will examine each superfood in greater detail, looking at their individual advantages, suggested serving sizes, and novel methods to work them into our regular diets. Get ready to be amazed as we reveal the incredible power of these superfoods and how they may help us age gracefully and beautifully.

Definition of superfoods

There has been a surge in the use of the phrase "superfoods" in recent years, usually referring to a variety of foods that are particularly beneficial to one's health. Although the term "superfood" lacks a precise scientific meaning, it has come to be understood as referring to a certain class of foods that are exceptionally rich in beneficial nutrients and bioactive chemicals.

Vitamins, minerals, antioxidants, phytochemicals, and other useful compounds are abundant in superfoods, making them ideal for achieving and maintaining peak health. For individuals trying to get the most out of their calorie intake, they are a great option because of the high nutritious content per calorie.

The unique health advantages of superfoods come from the extremely high levels of certain nutrients and bioactive substances they contain. Antioxidants, which help prevent oxidative damage to our cells by neutralizing damaging free radicals, may be among these chemicals. Anti-inflammatory, anti-carcinogenic, and anti-aging phytochemicals are common in several superfoods.

Keep in mind that superfoods are not meant to substitute a healthy, well-rounded diet, nor are they a magic bullet. Instead, they should be considered part of a balanced and varied diet. When added to a diet that also includes other nutrient-rich foods, superfoods can provide an additional nutritional boost and aid in overall health.

Fruits and vegetables, whole grains, nuts and seeds, legumes, and fish are all examples of superfoods. Each "superfood" has its own special collection of nutrients and health advantages. Berries, for instance, provide a lot of beneficial antioxidants, greens are loaded with nutrients, and seafood is a good source of healthy omega-3 fatty acids. The best way to get all the nutrients we need is to eat a wide range of superfoods.

It's important to note that just because something is labeled a "superfood" doesn't mean you can pig yourself on it without thinking about your calorie count or the rest of your diet. Consuming superfoods as part of a healthy diet that also contains other sources of essential nutrients is optimal. The benefits of superfoods are maximized when they are consumed with moderation and variety.

Local and regional cuisine have been shown to have significant health benefits and should not be neglected. Superfoods can come from any food, anywhere in the globe; they are not confined to rare or expensive products. The goal is to eat a wide variety of meals that are both high in nutrients and enjoyable to one's particular palate and cultural background.

Foods that are considered "superfoods" have a high concentration of beneficial nutrients and bioactive substances and, as a result, provide extraordinary health advantages. You can improve your health and well-being by include them in your diet. Maximizing the nutritional content of our diet and aiding our pursuit of bright and optimal health can be accomplished by include a wide range of superfoods in our daily fare. Keep in mind that the synergy of a varied and balanced diet is what truly nourishes our bodies and encourages longevity, not just the sum of their superfood parts.

The role of antioxidants in aging

There is a complicated interplay between genetic predisposition, lifestyle choices, and environmental influences that contribute to the aging process. The imbalance between the generation of free radicals and the body's ability to neutralize them is called oxidative stress, and it is widely recognized as a substantial contributor to the aging process. Damage to cells, faster aging, and an uptick in the chance of developing chronic diseases are all possible outcomes of this discord. Antioxidants have a role in this context.

Antioxidants are substances that can neutralize free radicals and reduce the harmful consequences of oxidative stress. They protect our cells and DNA by canceling out the effects of free radicals. Antioxidants assist maintain a healthy internal environment by defending against the damaging effects of oxidative stress.

Antioxidants play an important part in aging, but their effects go far beyond cellular wellness. Some of the most important roles that antioxidants play in promoting healthy aging are as follows:

Cellular health

DNA, proteins, and lipids are all susceptible to damage from free radicals. This impairment in cellular communication and function can raise the risk of developing age-related illnesses. By neutralizing free radicals, antioxidants help prevent or lessen the severity of this damage, benefiting our cells' health and functionality.

Skin health

Constant exposure to UV light and pollutants, for example, can cause free radical production and hasten the skin's aging process. Oxidative stress, inflammation, and collagen synthesis can all be prevented, mitigated, or supported by antioxidant use either topically or orally. This has the potential to boost skin health, slow the aging process, and make you look younger.

Cognitive function

Cognitive decline and neurodegenerative illnesses like Alzheimer's and Parkinson's are linked to oxidative stress and inflammation. Supporting brain health and cognitive function may be possible with the help of antioxidants, especially those with anti-inflammatory characteristics. They promote healthy brain aging, decrease brain inflammation, and protect neurons from injury.

Cardiovascular health

The role of oxidative stress in the onset and progression of cardiovascular illnesses is central. Antioxidants have been proven to aid in vascular health maintenance, inflammation reduction, and LDL cholesterol oxidation prevention, all of which play a role in atherosclerosis formation. Antioxidants help the heart stay healthy and age gracefully by lowering inflammation and oxidative stress.

Overall disease prevention

Increased oxidative stress and inflammation are typically linked to the development of chronic diseases like cancer, diabetes, and cardiovascular disease. Antioxidants' anti-inflammatory and free radical-scavenging properties also make them useful for preventing certain conditions. Antioxidants aid in healthy aging by bolstering general health and warding off the advent of chronic diseases.

Antioxidants are extremely helpful in maintaining healthy aging, but they are not a miracle cure. Antioxidants' efficacy in the body is affected by a number of variables, such as their bioavailability, interactions with other nutrients, and metabolic differences between people. Therefore, rather than relying entirely on supplements, it is preferable to receive antioxidants through a diversified and balanced diet.

One preventative and all-natural way to promote good aging is to eat foods high in antioxidants. Antioxidants can be found in abundance in foods with vibrant colors. This includes berries, leafy greens, tomatoes, and citrus fruits, to name a few. Nuts, seeds, whole grains, and spices like turmeric and cinnamon are all good options.

By scavenging harmful free radicals, decreasing oxidative stress, and bolstering cellular and systemic health,

3-44

antioxidants significantly contribute to the promotion of healthy aging. Consuming a diet high in antioxidant-rich foods has been shown to slow down the aging process, increase longevity, and improve quality of life in old age.

List of superfoods and their benefits

Superfoods are an impressive category of foods that are both high in nutrients and low in calories. The addition of these items to our diets can provide a boost of vital nutrients, antioxidants, and bioactive chemicals that are beneficial to our health in general. Let's have a look at a few examples of famous superfoods and the benefits they provide:

Berries

Blueberries, strawberries, and raspberries are just a few examples of berries that are high in fiber, vitamin C, and antioxidants. They're linked to a healthier brain, body, and blood sugar level as well as better cardiovascular health and lower inflammation.

Leafy greens

Nutritionally, dark green leafy vegetables like spinach, kale, and Swiss chard are unparalleled. They help maintain strong bones and hearts, aid in detoxifying, and supply vital minerals.

Seeds and nuts

Healthy fats, fiber, and nutrients galore may all be found in nuts and seeds including almonds, walnuts, chia seeds, and flaxseeds. They have antioxidant and anti-inflammatory effects, help with weight management, improve heart health, and deliver brain-boosting omega-3 fatty acids.

Fish oils

Omega-3 fatty acids, found in abundance in oily fish like salmon, sardines, and mackerel, have anti-inflammatory effects and are good for heart health, brain function, and skin health. In addition, they supply vital nutrients and high-quality protein.

Turmeric

Curcumin, found in the spice turmeric, is an effective antioxidant and anti-inflammatory agent. It may provide protection against chronic diseases including cancer and heart disease and has been linked to decreased inflammation, better brain health, and increased immunological function.

Green tea

Catechins, the antioxidants found in abundance in green tea, have been linked to a variety of health advantages. Consumption of green tea has been linked to better cognitive performance, weight control, lower risk of cardiovascular disease and some cancers, and a faster metabolic rate.

Dark chocolate

High-cocoa-content dark chocolate is an excellent source of antioxidants and flavonoids. Clinical trials have indicated that it improves cardiovascular health by reducing blood pressure, inflammation, and cholesterol levels. There's some evidence that eating dark chocolate can improve your mood and keep your brain healthy.

Greek yogurt

Greek yogurt has many health benefits, including a high protein content, probiotics, calcium, and other minerals. It helps the digestive system work better, makes you feel fuller for longer, and is good for your bones.

Quinoa

Protein, fiber, and minerals like magnesium and iron may all be found in quinoa, making it a highly nutritious grain. It is gluten-free, has a high digestibility rate, and a full complement of amino acids. Quinoa helps with weight loss, keeps you feeling full longer, and is good for your heart.

Avocado

The monounsaturated fats, fiber, vitamins, and minerals included in avocados are beneficial to heart health. It helps keep your mind sharp, your skin and hair healthy, your waistline trim, and it even has antioxidant and anti-inflammatory benefits.

Tomatoes

Lycopene, a potent antioxidant, is responsible for the deep red color of tomatoes. Certain types of cancer, heart disease, and eye disorders may be prevented by eating foods rich in lycopene. In addition to vitamin C and potassium, tomatoes also contain other healthy nutrients.

Legumes

Chickpeas, lentils, and black beans are just a few examples of legumes that are high quality plant-based protein, fiber, and nutritional sources. They are beneficial to one's cardiovascular system, digestive system, weight, and energy levels.

Keep in mind that these superfoods will work best as part of a well-rounded diet that also contains a wide array of other nutrient-dense foods. Maximizing health benefits and ensuring a wide range of critical nutrients, variety is the key.

There are many easy ways to incorporate superfoods into our diets, such as adding berries to our morning oatmeal, leafy greens to our salads, nuts as a snack, a cup of green tea after a meal, or trying out new dishes that highlight these nutrient powerhouses.

Superfoods provide a wealth of beneficial nutrients, antioxidants, and bioactive substances that contribute to our health, speed up the aging process, and improve our quality of life.

4. The Power of Supplements

5. Clean Living for a Healthier Future

Welcoming you to the enlightened world of clean living, where we will investigate the life-altering potential of deliberate decisions that benefit our health, happiness, and the planet. In this chapter, we will investigate what it means to live a clean lifestyle, why it's important, what it takes to make the transition, and what effect it has on how we age. Prepare to set out on a path of environmentally responsible decisions and learn how a green lifestyle can lead to a better, longer life.

The term "clean living" refers to a way of life that takes into account the effects our actions will have on our bodies, minds, and the environment as a whole. Toxin-free living is the deliberate selection of goods, procedures, and routines that do not contain or produce hazardous toxins, chemicals, or pollutants. What we eat, what we use, and the decisions we make about our waste and environmental effect are all part of what it means to live a clean lifestyle.

Cleanliness is of paramount importance. Toxins and pollutants, which can have negative impacts on human health, are becoming increasingly common in today's environment. Pesticides in food, chemicals in cleaning supplies, and environmental pollutants can all build up in people over time and exacerbate preexisting conditions. By adopting eco-friendly lifestyles, we protect ourselves and future generations from unnecessary exposure to toxic chemicals.

Keeping clean doesn't have to be a difficult or time-consuming process. Making deliberate decisions and changing over to more eco-friendly practices is what "clean living" is all about.

Living a healthy, clean lifestyle has a significant effect on how quickly you age. Toxin reduction and an overall cleaner lifestyle can help us keep our bodies in top shape as we become older.

To assist you apply clean living ideas into your daily life, we will go deeper into these concrete ways of living in the following sections of this chapter. The healthier and more sustainable future we and future generations may create is one that embraces clean living.

Definition and importance of clean living

Clean living is a way of life that emphasizes making and engaging in decisions and routines that are beneficial to one's health, happiness, and the long-term viability of the planet. Making lifestyle changes that reduce our exposure to potentially dangerous substances, poisons, and pollutants in our immediate surroundings and beyond is an important part of being environmentally conscious. What we eat, what we use, what we breathe, and how we affect the environment are all part of what constitutes a "clean" lifestyle.

Responsibility for one's own health and the planet's is at the heart of the "clean living" movement. It involves being aware of the effects our actions have on ourselves, others, and the world around us, and choosing actions that do less damage and contribute more to our well-being.

Toxins, synthetic chemicals, and other potentially dangerous things are given little to no priority in a clean lifestyle. It promotes the consumption of food and other items that haven't been chemically altered in any way. This is true of many things we put into our bodies and into our houses, including the food we eat, the personal care items we use, the cleaning agents we employ, and the building materials we select.

Cleanliness is of paramount importance. Toxins and pollutants abound in today's contemporary society, and they can have serious consequences for human health. Allergies, hormone disruptions, respiratory troubles, and even chronic diseases have all been linked to the accumulation of toxic compounds in the body, caused by everything from the chemicals in our cleaning goods and personal care items to the air pollution we breathe every day.

Adopting a more eco-friendly lifestyle means taking measures to lessen our contact with potentially dangerous chemicals, making the world a better place for current and future generations. There are several advantages to leading a clean lifestyle, such as:

Improved personal health

A reduction in one's exposure to potentially dangerous chemicals and poisons is one of the goals of "clean living practices," which emphasize the use of natural and organic products. This, in turn, can benefit health in many ways, including the respiratory system, the immune system, hormone balance, and general well-being.

Reduced toxic load

The goal of a "clean lifestyle" is to reduce one's contact with the many sources of pollution and toxicity one encounters on a daily basis. By making non-toxic substitutions, we lessen the toxic burden on our bodies, improving the health of our organs and systems and decreasing the likelihood of developing chronic diseases.

Environmental sustainability

The benefits of a healthy lifestyle extend beyond one's own body to include the health of the planet. Reduced plastic use, energy conservation, and consumer support for ethical and environmentally conscious firms are all examples of eco-friendly and sustainable actions that help protect the planet's natural resources for future generations.

Mind-body connection

The importance of our mental and physical health being intertwined is emphasized by a life of cleanliness. Maintaining a clean and orderly home, a regular exercise routine, a focus on the present moment, and a diet rich in nutritious foods all contribute to our mental and emotional wellness.

Long-term benefits

Living a clean lifestyle is preventative and beneficial in the long run. We may improve our health, longevity, and happiness by making clean living choices early in life and sticking to them throughout our lives.

The term "clean living" refers to a way of life that prioritizes making ethical decisions, restricts one's intake of potentially harmful substances, and prioritizes one's own health and the health of the planet. Well-being, less exposure to hazardous substances, and future sustainability are all gained through the adoption of clean living practices. The goal of a healthy, sustainable lifestyle is not perfection but rather the conscious adoption of practices that benefit both the individual and the earth.

Practical ways to live clean

Living a clean lifestyle is not about perfection or drastic changes. It's about making conscious choices and gradually adopting practices that prioritize our health and minimize our impact on the environment. Here are some practical ways to embrace clean living in everyday life:

Non-toxic home products
Cleaning products

Replace conventional cleaning products, which often contain harsh chemicals, with non-toxic alternatives. Look for natural or eco-friendly options that use plant-based ingredients and are free from harmful substances like ammonia, chlorine, and phthalates. Alternatively, you can make your own cleaning solutions using ingredients like vinegar, baking soda, lemon juice, and essential oils.

Personal care products

Many personal care products, such as soaps, shampoos, and cosmetics, contain synthetic ingredients that can be harmful to both our health and the environment. Opt for natural and organic alternatives that are free from harmful additives like parabens, sulfates, and artificial fragrances. Look for products with simple, recognizable ingredients and certifications such as USDA organic or cruelty-free.

Indoor air quality

Improve indoor air quality by reducing exposure to indoor pollutants. Choose low or zero VOC (volatile organic compound) paints and finishes when decorating or renovating your home. Consider using air purifiers or indoor plants that can help filter and purify the air. Regularly open windows to allow fresh air to circulate and remove indoor pollutants.

Choosing organic and natural foods

Organic produce

Opt for organic fruits and vegetables whenever possible. Organic farming practices reduce exposure to synthetic pesticides, fertilizers, and genetically modified organisms (GMOs). These foods are not only healthier for us but also support sustainable farming methods that are better for the environment.

Whole, unprocessed foods

Focus on whole, unprocessed foods that are as close to their natural state as possible. Choose fresh fruits and vegetables, whole grains, lean proteins, and healthy fats. Minimize consumption of highly processed foods that often contain additives, preservatives, and artificial ingredients.

Read labels

Be mindful of food labels and ingredient lists. Avoid products with excessive added sugars, artificial sweeteners, hydrogenated oils, and other unhealthy additives. Look for foods with minimal, recognizable ingredients and opt for products made with organic, non-GMO, and sustainable ingredients.

Reducing plastic use

Bring your own reusable bags

Instead of using plastic bags at the grocery store, bring your own reusable bags made from cloth or sturdy materials. Keep a few bags in your car or carry a foldable one in your bag for unexpected shopping trips.

Choose reusable water bottles

Invest in a reusable water bottle made from stainless steel, glass, or BPA-free plastic. Fill it with filtered tap water instead of purchasing single-use plastic bottles. If you're concerned about water quality, consider using a home water filtration system.

Say no to single-use plastics

Reduce your use of single-use plastics like straws, utensils, and food containers. Carry reusable alternatives such as stainless steel straws, bamboo utensils, and glass or stainless-steel food containers. When dining out, kindly decline plastic straws or bring your own reusable one.

Bulk shopping and meal planning

Purchase food items in bulk to minimize packaging waste. Bring your own reusable containers to fill with bulk items like grains, nuts, and dried fruits. Plan your meals and snacks ahead of time to reduce the need for individually packaged convenience foods.

By implementing these practical steps, you can gradually reduce your exposure to toxins, promote a healthier lifestyle, and minimize your environmental footprint. Remember, living clean is a journey, and small changes can make a significant impact over time.

Impact of clean living on aging process

Clean living practices can have a significant impact on the aging process, promoting vitality, longevity, and overall well-being. By adopting a clean lifestyle, we reduce our exposure to harmful substances, prioritize our health, and support our bodies in aging gracefully. Here are some ways in which clean living can positively influence the aging process:

Enhanced cellular health

Clean living practices, such as consuming organic and natural foods, provide our bodies with essential nutrients and antioxidants necessary for cellular health. Nutrient-dense foods rich in vitamins, minerals, and phytochemicals nourish our cells and support their optimal function. Antioxidants help protect our cells from damage caused by free radicals, reducing oxidative stress and supporting healthy aging.

Improved gut health

Clean living emphasizes the consumption of whole, unprocessed foods and the avoidance of artificial additives and preservatives. By choosing organic and natural foods, we support our gut health, which plays a crucial role in nutrient absorption, immune function, and overall well-being. A healthy gut microbiome contributes to a strong immune system, improved digestion, and a reduced risk of age-related diseases.

Reduced inflammation

Inflammation is a natural response of the immune system, but chronic inflammation can contribute to the aging process and the development of chronic diseases. Clean living practices, such as consuming anti-inflammatory foods and avoiding pro-inflammatory substances, help reduce inflammation in the body. A diet rich in fruits, vegetables, whole grains, and healthy fats can support a balanced inflammatory response, promoting overall health and longevity.

Skin health

Clean living practices can have a positive impact on skin health and the aging of our largest organ. By choosing natural and non-toxic skincare products, we reduce the risk of skin irritations, sensitivities, and exposure to harmful chemicals. Consuming a clean diet rich in antioxidants, healthy fats, and hydration supports skin health from within. It can help reduce the appearance of wrinkles, promote a youthful glow, and support overall skin integrity.

Mental and emotional well-being

Clean living practices extend beyond the physical realm and also encompass mental and emotional well-being. Engaging in regular exercise, practicing stress management techniques, and cultivating a positive mindset all contribute to healthy aging. Exercise promotes brain health, reduces the risk of cognitive decline, and improves mood and overall well-being. Stress management techniques, such as mindfulness and meditation, help reduce stress levels, support mental clarity, and promote a sense of calm and balance.

By embracing clean living practices, we prioritize our health, support our bodies in aging well, and create a foundation for a vibrant and fulfilling life. Clean living is not about perfection but rather making conscious choices that align with our values and promote overall well-being. With each clean living step we take, we contribute to a healthier and more vibrant future, not only for ourselves but for future generations as well.

6. The Influence of Physical Activity

Welcome to the captivating world of physical activity and its profound impact on both the body and mind. In this chapter, we will explore the numerous benefits of regular exercise, including its positive effects on physical health, mental well-being, and the aging process. Get ready to discover the transformative power of movement and uncover the various forms of exercise that can enhance your overall well-being.

Regular exercise is not only vital for maintaining a healthy weight and improving physical fitness, but it also offers a wide range of benefits for our mental and emotional well-being. Engaging in physical activity has been linked to reduced stress levels, improved mood, increased energy, enhanced cognitive function, and a lower risk of developing chronic diseases. It is a powerful tool that can improve our quality of life and contribute to healthy aging.

Incorporating physical activity into our daily routine doesn't have to be daunting. Remember to listen to your body and choose activities that suit your fitness level and abilities. If you have any health concerns, consult with a healthcare professional before starting a new exercise program.

In the following sections of this chapter, we will dive deeper into the specific benefits of each form of exercise and provide practical tips for incorporating physical activity into your daily routine. By embracing regular exercise, you can unlock the incredible benefits it offers and experience the transformative power of movement on your journey to holistic well-being.

Benefits of regular exercise to body and mind

Regular exercise is a powerful tool that offers a multitude of benefits for both the body and mind. Engaging in physical activity on a consistent basis has a profound impact on our overall well-being and contributes to healthy aging. Let's explore some of the key benefits that regular exercise provides:

Physical health benefits

Weight management

Regular exercise plays a crucial role in weight management by burning calories and increasing metabolism. It helps maintain a healthy body weight and reduce the risk of obesity, which is linked to numerous chronic diseases.

Cardiovascular health

Engaging in aerobic exercises, such as brisk walking, jogging, or cycling, improves cardiovascular health. It strengthens the heart muscle, increases lung capacity, and improves circulation. Regular aerobic exercise can lower the risk of heart disease, reduce blood pressure, improve cholesterol levels, and enhance overall cardiovascular fitness.

Strong muscles and bones

Strength training exercises, such as lifting weights or using resistance bands, promote the development of strong muscles and bones. As we age, maintaining muscle mass and bone density becomes increasingly important. Regular strength training can help prevent muscle loss, improve bone density, and reduce the risk of osteoporosis and fractures.

Enhanced immune function

Regular exercise has been shown to enhance immune function, reducing the risk of illness and infection. It can strengthen the immune system by promoting the circulation of immune cells, increasing the body's defense against pathogens, and reducing inflammation.

Improved energy levels

Engaging in physical activity boosts energy levels by increasing blood flow, delivering oxygen and nutrients to the body's tissues. Regular exercise improves stamina, reduces fatigue, and promotes overall vitality and energy levels.

Mental and emotional well-being

Reduced stress and anxiety

Exercise has a profound impact on mental health by reducing stress and anxiety levels. Physical activity stimulates the production of endorphins, neurotransmitters that promote feelings of happiness and well-being. Regular exercise can act as a natural stress reliever and improve mood.

Improved cognitive function

Physical activity has been linked to improved cognitive function, including enhanced memory, attention, and problem-solving skills. Exercise promotes the release of growth factors that help create new nerve cells and improve brain function.

Increased brain health

Regular exercise has been shown to protect against age-related cognitive decline and reduce the risk of neurodegenerative diseases such as Alzheimer's and dementia. It promotes better blood flow to the brain, increases the production of neuroprotective proteins, and enhances brain plasticity.

Better sleep quality

Regular exercise can improve sleep quality and promote restful sleep. It helps regulate the sleep-wake cycle, reduces insomnia symptoms, and enhances overall sleep duration and quality.

Enhanced mood and self-esteem

Engaging in physical activity boosts mood and self-esteem by promoting the release of endorphins, reducing symptoms of depression, and increasing self-confidence. Regular exercise can provide a sense of accomplishment, improve body image, and enhance overall well-being.

The benefits of regular exercise extend beyond the physical and mental realms, positively influencing various aspects of our lives. Whether it's improving physical fitness, reducing the risk of chronic diseases, boosting mood and self-esteem, or promoting healthy aging, exercise is a key component of a holistic approach to well-being.

It's important to note that the type and intensity of exercise should be tailored to individual abilities and health conditions. Before starting a new exercise program, it's advisable to consult with a healthcare professional or a qualified fitness instructor to ensure safety and suitability.

Various forms of exercises and their impact on aging

Regular exercise is essential for healthy aging, and incorporating different types of exercises into our routine can maximize the benefits. Let's explore three popular forms of exercise—cardiovascular exercises, strength training, and yoga and Pilates—and their specific impacts on aging:

Cardiovascular exercises

Cardiovascular exercises, also known as aerobic exercises, are activities that increase the heart rate and breathing rate, thereby improving cardiovascular health. They have numerous benefits for aging individuals:

Heart health

Cardiovascular exercises strengthen the heart muscle, improve blood circulation, and enhance the efficiency of the cardiovascular system. This reduces the risk of heart disease, lowers blood pressure, and improves overall cardiovascular fitness.

Weight management

Regular cardiovascular exercise helps maintain a healthy weight by burning calories and increasing metabolism. As we age, maintaining a healthy weight becomes increasingly important for preventing chronic diseases and promoting overall well-being.

Increased endurance and energy levels

Engaging in cardiovascular exercises boosts endurance and stamina, allowing older adults to maintain their energy levels for daily activities. It improves lung capacity and oxygen delivery to the muscles, making everyday tasks feel easier and reducing the risk of fatigue.

Improved brain health

Cardiovascular exercises increase blood flow to the brain, promoting the delivery of oxygen and nutrients. This enhances cognitive function, memory, and overall brain health, reducing the risk of age-related cognitive decline and neurodegenerative diseases.

Mental well-being

Cardiovascular exercises stimulate the release of endorphins, which are natural mood boosters. Regular participation in aerobic activities can reduce stress, anxiety, and symptoms of depression, improving mental well-being and promoting a positive outlook on life.

Strength training

Strength training involves using resistance, such as weights or resistance bands, to build muscle strength and endurance. It offers several unique benefits for aging individuals:

Increased muscle mass and bone density

As we age, we naturally lose muscle mass and bone density. Strength training helps counteract this decline by promoting muscle growth and bone remodeling. It improves overall strength, balance, and stability, reducing the risk of falls and fractures.

Metabolic boost
Strength training increases muscle mass, which in turn increases the body's metabolic rate. This helps older adults maintain a healthy weight and manage their metabolism effectively, reducing the risk of obesity and related chronic diseases.

Joint health and flexibility
Strength training exercises that involve full-body movements or specific joint exercises can improve joint health and flexibility. This enhances mobility, reduces joint pain, and promotes better overall physical function.

Enhanced independence and daily living activities
Strong muscles are essential for performing daily activities, such as carrying groceries, climbing stairs, or getting up from a chair. Strength training improves functional strength, making these activities easier and promoting independence as we age.

Hormonal benefits
Strength training can positively impact hormone levels in older adults. It can increase the production of growth hormone, which supports tissue repair, muscle growth, and

overall vitality. It also helps regulate hormones associated with mood, stress, and sleep, promoting overall well-being.

Yoga and Pilates

Yoga and Pilates are mind-body exercises that focus on flexibility, balance, and core strength. They offer unique benefits for aging individuals:

Improved flexibility and balance

Both yoga and Pilates emphasize stretching and gentle movements that promote flexibility and balance. This reduces the risk of falls, improves posture, and enhances overall mobility and physical function.

Enhanced mind-body connection

Yoga and Pilates incorporate breath control, mindfulness, and relaxation techniques. They promote a deep mind-body connection, reducing stress, improving mental focus, and enhancing overall well-being.

Core strength and stability

Both practices emphasize core engagement and development, which is crucial for maintaining a strong and stable body. A strong core improves posture, supports the spine, and reduces the risk of back pain.

Stress reduction and relaxation

Yoga and Pilates incorporate techniques such as deep breathing, meditation, and relaxation exercises, which promote stress reduction and relaxation. These practices can lower blood pressure, improve sleep quality, and enhance mental well-being.

Joint mobility and pain relief
The gentle, controlled movements in yoga and Pilates can help improve joint mobility and reduce joint pain. They provide a low-impact form of exercise that is accessible to individuals with joint conditions or limitations.

Incorporating a combination of cardiovascular exercises, strength training, and mind-body exercises like yoga and Pilates can provide a well-rounded exercise routine that addresses various aspects of physical fitness and promotes healthy aging. It's essential to consult with a healthcare professional or a qualified fitness instructor before starting a new exercise program, especially if you have any existing health conditions or concerns.

Suggestions for incorporating physical activity into daily routine

If you want to lead a healthy life and improve your general health, you need to make exercise a regular part of your schedule. Here are some doable tips to incorporate fitness into your daily routine:

Prioritize movement
Move more frequently and purposefully throughout the day. Always be on the lookout for ways to be involved, no matter

how tiny. Walk around the office for a few minutes every hour, stretch, and try to avoid sitting as much as possible. All these little things you do might add up to a significant amount of exercise.

Set achievable goals

To get started, you should make goals that are reasonable given your current fitness and lifestyle. Think practically about how much time and effort you can put into working out. Start with a manageable target, such as exercising for 30 minutes at a moderate effort most days of the week, and go up from there.

Find activities you enjoy

Pick out some physical pursuits that you'll look forward to doing. Participating in activities that you enjoy, such as dancing, swimming, cycling, hiking, or playing a sport, will make exercise more fun and enhance your motivation to keep it up. Try out a variety of pursuits to see what you enjoy doing.

Schedule dedicated exercise time

Make time in your schedule for exercise and honor it as if it were a mandatory meeting. Schedule in time for exercise the same way you would for any other major commitment. If you put in the time to exercise in your calendar, you'll be more likely to make it a priority.

Mix it up

Change up your routine to keep things interesting and give your body new challenges. Include in your regimen some aerobic activity, some strength training, and some activities that focus on your flexibility. This way, you can be confident that you're improving your fitness in all areas, and it also keeps things interesting. If you're looking to mix up your exercise routine, try something new by enrolling in a class, joining a club, or consulting a website for a workout.

Make it social

Join a group fitness class or work out with a friend to turn exercise into something fun to do together. Motivation, accountability, and a feeling of belonging can all be gained by working out with a friend or joining a club. It can also increase your motivation and make workout more pleasurable.

Break it up

If it's hard for you to set aside significant periods of time for exercise, try breaking up your routine into multiple shorter sessions spread out throughout the day. You can take a yoga session in the evening, go for a 10-minute walk in the morning, and perform a 15-minute strength training workout during the day. More beneficial than one long workout is a series of shorter ones.

Incorporate physical activity into daily tasks

Actively seek out activities you can do throughout the day. If your errand is short, maybe you might walk or ride your bike there instead of driving. Instead of taking the elevator or escalator, walk up the steps. Put some distance between your automobile and your destination so you can walk more. Making even a few of these adjustments can have a cumulative effect and get you moving more.

Make it a family affair

Encourage physical activity among family members. Organize some outdoor activities for the weekend that everyone can take part in. Involving those you care about most can make exercising more enjoyable and more of a habit for everyone involved.

Monitor your progress

Record your workouts and track your improvement. Track your workouts, steps, and other forms of exercise with a fitness tracker or a smartphone app. Keeping track of your successes can give you a sense of pride and fulfillment, which helps keep you focused on your mission.

Always go at a pace that feels good to you, and work your way up to a higher intensity and longer workout. Talk to your doctor before beginning an exercise routine if you have any preexisting conditions or haven't been active in a while.

There are many positive effects on your body, mood, and mind when you make exercise a regular part of your life. It will help you get in shape, feel better emotionally, have more stamina, and age gracefully. Enjoy the process and make physical activity a staple in your life.

7.   *The Role of Mental Well-being in Aging*

This chapter explores the correlation between mental health and the natural aging process, and offers advice on how to take good care of your mind at any age. Learn the life-altering effects of a good outlook on aging, stress management, cognitive exercises, and more.

The state of one's mind is an important indicator of general health and has a profound impact on how we age. All of these things, and more, are affected by our mental health. Through self-awareness and care, we may strengthen our mental health, keep our minds sharp, keep our emotions in check, and age with dignity and zest.

We will uncover the impact that our mental health has on numerous elements of our lives as we age and examine the significant relationship between the two in the following sections. We'll look into workouts and methods proven to improve mental health as we age, boosting brain power, mood, and contentment. We'll also talk about how keeping a positive outlook has been shown to slow down the aging process for some people.

Understanding the connection between mental health and aging

How we feel about becoming older is heavily influenced by our mental health, so understanding the link between the two is essential. The state of our minds has a profound impact on our ability to learn and remember new information, how we feel emotionally and socially, how we relate to others, and how long we can expect to live. Let's dive deeper into the significance of the age-related decline in mental health:

Cognitive function

The state of one's mind and their ability to think clearly are inextricably linked. Taking care of one's mental health benefits one's overall cognitive functioning, boosting things like memory, focus, and problem solving. The risk of cognitive decline and dementia is increased in people with mental health problems such as depression, anxiety, or chronic stress. Maintaining one's mental health in a variety of ways is associated with better cognitive function and a longer, more fulfilling life in old age.

Emotional well-being

Our emotional well-being is profoundly affected by our mental health. Changes in our physical and mental health, as well as the passing of loved ones, can all have an effect on how we feel as we become older. Emotional resilience is bolstered by good mental health, making it easier to deal with adversity while keeping a positive view. When mental health issues aren't addressed, though, they can cause suffering, worse quality of life, and even social isolation. Emotional health and longevity can be improved by making self-care for the mind a priority and reaching out for help when it's needed.

Social interactions and relationships

Maintaining positive mental health is essential for fostering fulfilling relationships as we become older. Taking care of one's mental health is important for many reasons, including but not limited to: making and keeping friends; participating in community activities; and feeling accepted and loved. On the flip side, mental illness can cause people to withdraw from others and cause friction in existing relationships. Focusing on one's mental health allows one to invest in one's relationships, leading to a more full and robust existence.

Resilience and adaptation

The state of one's mental health has an effect on one's resiliency in the face of adversity. Adapting to bodily changes, retirement, or new responsibilities is a common part of the aging process. Having a healthy mind helps us adapt to changing circumstances and move on with optimism and grace. However, unaddressed mental health disorders can impede adjustment to new circumstances and heighten emotional strain and difficulties coping. Taking care of one's mental health in a variety of ways makes it possible to accept the inevitable changes that occur with becoming older and to persevere when faced with adversity.

Overall quality of life

The quality of our lives as we become older is greatly influenced by our mental health. Increased contentment, joy, and fulfillment in life are the results of caring for and giving attention to one's mental health. Taking care of one's mental health has beneficial effects on one's physical health, relationships, and ability to participate in things that matter to one. A robust and meaningful life, full of purpose and joy, can be cultivated by prioritizing mental health as we age.

Recognizing the close relationship between mental health and longevity highlights the significance of giving our mental health the attention it deserves at all stages of life. We may improve our general health and accept aging with poise and resilience if we adopt techniques that assist mental health, such as mindfulness, cognitive exercises, stress management, and keeping a positive frame of mind. In the following paragraphs, we'll discuss methods for improving our mental health that can help us maintain a high quality of life as we get older.

Techniques for mental health care

Mindfulness and meditation

Mindfulness and meditation are potent methods for promoting emotional and psychological well-being. These methods encourage a mindful, nonjudgmental awareness of the internal and external experiences that make up the here and now. In this way, mindfulness and meditation benefit psychological well-being:

Stress reduction

Both mindfulness and meditation have been shown to be effective stress relievers. Present-moment awareness and emotional and mental neutrality are key components in developing serenity and contentment inside ourselves. Stress hormone levels can be lowered, emotional regulation can be strengthened, and resistance to stressors can be improved with consistent practice.

Improved emotional well-being

The techniques of mindfulness and meditation aid in the maturation of self-awareness and emotional control. They promote self-compassion and emotional resilience by letting us view our thoughts and feelings objectively and without judgment. By doing this on a regular basis, we can train ourselves to feel better emotionally.

Enhanced cognitive function

Studies have shown that mental abilities including attention, memory, and executive function can all benefit from regular mindfulness and meditation practice. Training one's attention on the here and now has been linked to gains in both cognitive performance and mental clarity.

Increased self-awareness

Meditation and other forms of mindfulness training might help you gain insight into yourself. The more we pay attention to our inner world—our thoughts, feelings, and body sensations—the more we learn about who we are and how we think and behave. Possessing this kind of insight is important for our mental health because it enables us to make deliberate decisions and respond to challenging situations with maturity and maturity.

Improved sleep quality

Better sleep quality has been linked to regular mindfulness and meditation practices. These methods can help alleviate insomnia by preparing the body and mind for a restful night's sleep. The mental health and well-being of an individual can benefit from better sleep.

Cognitive exercises

Mental acuity and efficiency can be enhanced through participation in cognitive exercises. Cognitive exercises, when practiced on a regular basis, can help preserve and even improve mental faculties as we age. Here are some brain-boosting activities:

Puzzles and brain games

Crossword puzzles, Sudoku, word searches, and brain-training apps are all great ways to exercise your brain and get better at solving problems. Doing things like this keeps the brain active and healthy.

Learning new skills

Playing an instrument, studying a new language, or picking up a new pastime are all great ways to challenge your brain and encourage neuroplasticity since they require you to learn new abilities. It improves brainpower by fortifying and establishing new connections between neurons.

Reading and mental stimulation

Keep your mind busy and fresh by reading on a regular basis, having mentally challenging conversations, or learning about new topics through reading, articles, or movies. Curiosity is piqued, critical thinking is encouraged, and chances for lifelong learning are presented through these exercises.

Memory exercises

Memory exercises, such as learning to memorize lists or sequences of numbers, or playing memory games, can help people retain and recall more information. Cognitive health can be improved through participation in these games.

Problem-solving and strategic games

Mental agility and the ability to make quick decisions are both enhanced by playing games like chess, Sudoku, and strategy video games. These kinds of exercises are great for maintaining mental flexibility.

Stress management

Techniques to effectively manage stress are essential for keeping one's mental health in good shape. Negative effects on mental health and the emergence of additional health problems are possible outcomes of prolonged exposure to stress. Methods to alleviate stress include the following:

Relaxation techniques

Deep breathing exercises, gradual muscular relaxation, and guided visualization are all examples of relaxation treatments that might assist trigger this physiological reaction. These methods help you relax and unwind by releasing built-up stress and muscle tension.

Physical activity

Walking, jogging, or practicing yoga on a regular basis is not only good for your health, but also helps you cope with stress. Endorphins are substances produced by the body during exercise that improve mood and assist lower stress and anxiety levels.

Time management and prioritization
Time management and setting priorities are two stress-busting strategies. Creating a more balanced and less stressful existence is possible through the use of techniques such as breaking down large activities into smaller, more manageable ones, creating achievable goals, and putting up protective barriers.

Social support
One effective strategy for handling stress is to reach out for help from those you care about. In trying circumstances, it might be helpful to talk about how you're feeling, ask for help or advice, or even just have someone listen.

Mind-body practices
Mind-body activities like yoga, tai chi, and qigong are excellent ways to improve your health and happiness. Stress is reduced through these activities, which mix light movement with attention to the breath.

Healthy lifestyle choices
One way to better handle stress is to adopt a healthy lifestyle, which includes eating right, exercising regularly, getting enough sleep, and cutting back on alcoholic beverages and

caffeine. Taking care of one's body strengthens one's mind and increases one's capacity for resilience.

Mindfulness and meditation activities, cognitive exercises, and methods for dealing with stress are all potent instruments for fostering mental health. We may improve our mental agility, lower our stress levels, and foster an optimistic outlook on life by incorporating these practices into our daily lives as we age. You may improve your mental health and quality of life significantly by adopting these habits as cornerstones of self-care.

The effect of a positive mindset on aging

A positive outlook is a valuable resource that can significantly affect how we age. The quality of our lives can be affected by the choices we make in terms of our thoughts, beliefs, and attitudes. Keeping a positive outlook can slow down the aging process in significant ways. Keeping an optimistic outlook has several advantages as we get older:

Physical health benefits

Numerous studies have shown that maintaining an optimistic outlook might have beneficial effects on one's physical well-being. Researchers have shown that people who have an optimistic attitude on life had fewer health problems and a longer life expectancy. It has been found to encourage healthy lifestyle choices that improve physical health, such as exercise, a nutritious diet, and enough of sleep.

Enhanced mental and emotional well-being

The state of one's mind and emotions can be greatly enhanced by adopting a more optimistic outlook. In addition to alleviating stress, worry, and depression, it also increases feelings of contentment, joy, and fulfillment. Maintaining emotional strength and resiliency requires keeping a positive attitude and dealing with life's setbacks as they arise.

Cognitive function and brain health

The cognitive benefits of maintaining an optimistic outlook have been well documented. Positive outlook has been linked to enhanced cognitive abilities such as working memory, flexibility, and executive control. Brain health, neuroplasticity, and longevity are all aided by maintaining an optimistic outlook on life.

Increased resilience and adaptability

We are better able to deal with the inevitable changes, difficulties, and losses that occur in life when we have an optimistic outlook. It allows us to see challenges not as insurmountable walls but as stepping stones on the path to success. This perspective helps us welcome transformation, adapt to new circumstances, and keep our spirits up in the face of setbacks.

Improved social relationships and connectedness

Positive thinking improves your ability to form bonds with others. As a result, it's simpler to meet new people and keep in touch with those you already have ties with. People who are optimistic are more likely to be kind, helpful, and supportive to those around them.

Increased motivation and goal attainment

A constructive outlook provides the fuel for motivation, which in turn propels us to realize our ambitions. Confidence in one's own abilities and a willingness to persevere in the face of adversity both increase when one adopts an optimistic worldview. The ability to focus, to overcome adversity, and to realize one's own potential are all facilitated by this uplifting inspiration.

Longer lifespan and healthy aging

Positive outlook has been linked to a longer life span and better aging, according to studies. Healthy lifestyle choices, a robust social network, and lower stress levels all lead to a longer life and higher quality of life for an optimistic person. By encouraging an optimistic and self-confident outlook, a positive frame of mind supports good aging.

Keeping a cheerful outlook is a skill that may be developed through time and supported in many ways. Examples of this category of items include:

Practicing gratitude

Positive thinking may flourish when we make it a habit to regularly show thanks for the good things in our life.

Challenging negative thoughts

Recognizing and questioning self-defeating ideas and assumptions might help you reframe things in a more constructive and liberating way.

Surrounding oneself with positive influences

Maintaining an optimistic outlook can be aided by surrounding oneself with positive, supportive people and participating in positive pursuits.

Engaging in self-care

Self-care, in the form of tending to one's health on all fronts (physical, emotional, and mental), is beneficial to one's state of mind and general happiness.

Practicing self-compassion

Self-compassion and self-kindness are powerful tools for building resilience and staying optimistic in the face of adversity.

Engaging in positive affirmations

A positive frame of mind can be strengthened through the use of positive affirmations, which can help to rewire our brains.

Aging positively allows us to view life with hope, resilience, and a belief in our own potential. As a result, we are better able to relish the good times, remain resilient in the face of adversity, and grow as people. The beauty and wisdom that come with age may only be appreciated if we maintain an optimistic outlook.

8. Sleep: The Underrated Elixir of Youth

The influence of sleep on our bodies and how we age is explored in this chapter. Uncovering the secrets of great sleep and providing practical strategies to optimize our sleep patterns, we explore the many positive benefits sleep has on our health and well-being.

The role of sleep in health and aging

The importance of sleep to our health and wellbeing increases with age. Some important facets of sleep's impact on health and longevity are as follows:

Physical restoration

While we snooze, our bodies restore and heal themselves. Growth hormones are secreted and healing of tissues and muscles takes place during this phase. Adequate sleep aids in physical recuperation, keeps immune system functioning at its best, and promotes general health and vitality.

Cognitive function

Brain health and restorative sleep go hand in hand. Memory, learning, and the capacity to solve problems are all helped along by it. Adequate sleep improves cognitive performance and productivity by fostering focus, imagination, and originality. However, chronic sleep loss has been linked to cognitive impairment, including memory and attentional problems.

Emotional well-being

The quality of our sleep greatly affects how we feel emotionally. We are better able to deal with stress, worry, and mood swings when we have had a restful night's sleep. Inadequate sleep, on the other hand, has been linked to heightened irritability, mood fluctuations, and the development of psychological disorders including melancholy and anxiety.

Hormonal balance

Sleep is essential for regulating the body's hormones. It aids in the maintenance of normal levels of hormones involved in the management of hunger, energy expenditure, and stress. Hormonal disruptions, such as those caused by interrupted sleep, have been linked to increased appetite, weight gain, and stress.

Cellular repair and aging

Healthy aging relies on regular sleep because it allows cells to repair and regenerate. While we are asleep, our bodies mend damaged cells and flush out harmful substances. Sleep deprivation has been linked to an accelerated aging process and an increase in the prevalence of age-related diseases.

Understanding the importance of sleep to our well-being as we age allows us to make it a priority in our lives. Sleeping regularly and getting enough sleep helps us feel better emotionally, perform better physically, and live longer. It helps us stay healthy and live longer, therefore it's important to any comprehensive strategy for improving our quality of life.

Techniques to improve sleep quality

Maximizing the recuperative effects of sleep requires enhancing its quality. Here are some easy things you may do to get better rest:

Establish a consistent sleep routine

Go to bed and get up at the same time every day, including on the weekends, and you'll have more control over your sleep schedule. Your internal clock will be better able to keep time and you'll have more regular sleep hours as a result.

Create a sleep-friendly environment

Create a space that allows you to relax and drift off to sleep easily. Your bedroom should be a calm, cool, and quiet place. Make sure you have a soft place to sleep, a supportive mattress and pillow, and as few distractions as possible, especially technological ones.

Practice good sleep hygiene

In order to teach your body that it's time to wind down and get ready for sleep, you need adopt some healthy sleep practices. Don't do anything mentally or visually engaging soon before bed. Start winding down for bed with a warm bath, a good book, or some deep breathing exercises.

Limit caffeine and alcohol intake

Both caffeine and alcohol have been shown to diminish the quality of sleep. Avoid drinking too close to bedtime, and especially in the evening, so that your body can relax on its own.

Create a technology-free zone

Limit your use of screens in the hour or so before up to bedtime, especially cellphones, tablets, and televisions. The hormone melatonin governs sleep, and exposure to the blue light emitted by these devices can interfere with its production. Make your bedroom a tech-free zone to unwind and cut back on screen time before night.

Manage stress

Anxiety and stress can make it difficult to get a good night's rest. Relax your body and mind with some deep breathing exercises, some mindfulness training, or writing down your thoughts before bed. Making these practices part of your nightly routine before bed can help you unwind and get some shut-eye.

Regular exercise

Better sleep quality is one of the many benefits of regular exercise. Exercise has been shown to improve sleep quality, but it's best to avoid doing it too soon to bedtime because of the stimulating effect it may have. Maintain a moderate exercise routine seven days a week, aiming for at least 30 minutes on most days.

Create a comfortable sleep environment

Make sure you have a peaceful, relaxing place to sleep. Think about the comfort of your sleeping environment, from temperature and noise to mattress and pillow firmness. Try out several blankets and pillows, and play around with the room's temperature and lighting until you find what works best for you.

Avoid large meals and excessive fluids before bed

Consuming a large meal or drinking too much liquid right before bed might cause pain and make it difficult to fall asleep. If you want to get a good night's sleep without being woken up by trips to the bathroom, it's best to go for light, balanced meals and restrict fluid intake in the evening.

Seek professional help if needed

If you have tried healthy sleep practices but are still having trouble falling or staying asleep, you may want to consult a medical expert. They can assess your sleeping habits, offer advice, and suggest treatments to help you get better rest.

You can improve your sleep quality, develop restful sleep routines, and make your bedroom more conducive to sleeping by using some or all of the following strategies. Raising the standard of one's slumber has a multiplicative effect on health, happiness, and success in all areas of life.

Addressing common sleep issues

Many people have trouble falling asleep or staying asleep, which can have a negative impact on their rest. In order to encourage comfortable and rejuvenating sleep, it is essential to address several common sleep difficulties. Some solutions to frequent sleeping problems are as follows:

Insomnia

The inability to fall asleep or remain asleep characterizes insomnia. Insomnia can be treated by committing to a regular sleep schedule, improving sleep hygiene, and developing a soothing pre-bedtime ritual. Reduce the number of naps you take during the day, limit stimulating activities or devices before night, and make your bedroom more conducive to sleep. Cognitive behavioral therapy for insomnia (CBT-I) is an option to consider if insomnia persists, or you can seek advice from a healthcare practitioner.

Sleep apnea

Sleep apnea is a sleep disorder in which breathing is repeatedly interrupted throughout the night, leading to restless sleep and excessive drowsiness throughout the day. Sleep apnea should be diagnosed and treated by a medical expert if it is suspected. Continuous positive airway pressure (CPAP) therapy, behavioral modification, and the use of oral devices are all viable options for treatment.

Restless legs syndrome (RLS)

In RLS, a person experiences an irresistible need to move their legs, which is typically accompanied by leg pain or other unpleasant symptoms. Establishing a regular sleep regimen, exercising regularly (but not right before bed), and avoiding caffeine and nicotine are all helpful in controlling RLS. If you need further diagnosis or treatment, see a doctor.

Shift work sleep disorder

The body's natural sleep-wake cycle can be severely disrupted by working shifts, making it difficult to fall asleep or stay asleep at the optimal times. Strategies to notify the body that it is time to sleep, such as wearing dark glasses on the way home from work to decrease exposure to sunshine, can help with shift work sleep problem management.

Anxiety and stress-related sleep issues

Trouble falling asleep or keeping asleep is a common complaint among those who regularly struggle with anxiety and stress. Deep breathing exercises, mindfulness meditation, and nightly journaling are just a few stress management strategies that might help you deal with these problems. Get into the habit of winding down before bed and making your bedroom a peaceful place to sleep. Seek expert assistance if stress and anxiety symptoms persist.

Environmental factors

The quality of your sleep may be compromised by environmental variables including noise, light, or an uncomfortable sleeping space. Reduce outside noise and light by utilizing earplugs, white noise generators, or blackout drapes. Make sure your bedroom is cool, has enough of ventilation, and has supportive bedding to help you get some shut-eye.

Medications and substances

The quality of your sleep may be negatively impacted by the use of certain drugs, caffeine, nicotine, and alcohol. Don't have any of those things right before bed. Talk to a doctor if you feel you need to explore other treatment options or make changes to your current prescription regimen.

Chronic pain

Sleep disturbances and insomnia are common complaints from those living with chronic pain. If you're having trouble sleeping due to chronic pain, try using pain management measures like heat or cold therapy, mild stretching before bed, or pain relievers. The best way to deal with chronic pain and get better rest is to go to a doctor.

Keep in mind that resolving sleep problems may call for specialized methods and expert advice. Give your sleep health top priority and get medical assistance if you need it. You can improve your health and longevity by preventing and treating common sleep disturbances so that you can enjoy restful, revitalizing sleep.

9. *Social Connections and Aging*

This chapter delves into the value of human connection, how to make and keep friends, and how to motivate people to get involved in their communities. Learn how forming and maintaining meaningful relationships can improve your quality of life, promote healthy aging, and fill you with happiness.

The impact of social interaction on aging

The way we interact with others has a significant impact on how we age. We're social creatures by design, so it's especially important to keep in touch with friends and family as we become older. Important facets of the effect of social interaction on aging are as follows:

Emotional well-being

Having meaningful relationships with other people is important to our mental health because it boosts our feelings of connectedness, safety, and acceptance. Loneliness and isolation can be overcome via social interaction, shared experiences, and a strong social network. A strong social network might help you feel less lonely, less stressed, and more optimistic.

Cognitive health

Better cognitive health and slower cognitive decline in old age have both been linked to regular social interaction. Keeping our minds active and alert requires us to interact with others in meaningful ways, such as through engaging discussion, enjoyable activities, and supportive social networks. Having meaningful relationships with other people is essential to keeping our brains healthy and our minds sharp.

Physical health

Physical well-being is also affected by people's social lives. Multiple studies have indicated that those who have close relationships with their friends and family tend to enjoy greater overall health. Lower rates of chronic diseases, lower risk of cardiovascular problems, and enhanced immunological function have all been linked to strong social relationships. Participating in social activities has been shown to improve adherence to healthful practices like exercise, a balanced diet, and medication.

Sense of purpose and fulfillment

We gain meaning and satisfaction through our relationships with other people. We feel a greater sense of purpose and belonging when we engage in meaningful relationships, make positive contributions to the lives of others, and participate actively in our communities. Motivation, a sense of self, and avenues for expansion and expression can all be discovered through interactions with others.

Mental well-being

The mental health benefits of socializing are well-documented. It aids in coping with adversity, lessens the likelihood of developing illnesses like depression and anxiety, and boosts one's psychological resilience in general. Feeling heard, acknowledged, and emotionally supported by others is a direct result of sharing our happiness, worries, and experiences with others.

Longevity and quality of life

Multiple studies have found that those who have close relationships with their friends and family have a higher life expectancy and a better quality of life overall. Social engagement promotes healthy aging and a higher quality of life in old age by providing emotional support, affection, and meaning.

The significance of fostering and maintaining social relationships as we age is highlighted by the recognition of the role that social interaction plays in the aging process. The tremendous benefits of social interaction can be experienced and a full and pleasant aging journey can be created via participation in social activities, the development of meaningful connections, and the promotion of a sense of community.

Cultivating and maintaining healthy relationships

To age in a healthy way, it is crucial to cultivate and sustain positive relationships with others. Here are some tried and true methods for keeping the bonds of love strong:

Active listening and empathy

Maintain an attitude of attentive listening in social interactions. Take an honest interest in what they have to say. You show that you care about and respect their opinion by listening to them carefully. Stronger relationships can be developed through the development of one's capacity for empathy.

Regular communication

Maintain constant lines of communication with your loved ones. Try to get in touch with them by setting up phone calls, video chats, or even face-to-face get-togethers. Plan get-togethers and outings to reconnect and keep the flame of your friendship burning.

Quality over quantity

Pay more attention to the depth of your connections than to their quantity. Focus on developing in-depth relationships with people that can add value to your life in terms of positivity, support, and personal development. Create bonds of happiness, contentment, and comprehension.

Shared activities and interests

Participate in group efforts and go after mutual goals. Do things that make you happy and put you in touch with people who share your interests. Participate in groups that share your interests, issues, or passions by joining a club or organization. Connections and shared memories are forged via shared experiences.

Give and receive support

When both parties are willing to put forth effort, the relationship grows stronger. Always be eager to help out and offer encouragement to those around you. Provide attentive listening, sound advice, and compassionate support at difficult circumstances. At the same time, it's important to let other people help you out. Putting yourself out there and being honest about your challenges will help build trust and closeness.

Embrace diversity

Connect with people who are different from you in age, culture, background, and viewpoint. Having meaningful interactions with people from different backgrounds helps you learn more about the world and yourself. Learn as much as you can from others and enjoy the enriched connections that result from their differences.

Practice forgiveness and let go of grudges

Conflict is inevitable in any relationship. Conflicts can be resolved via honest communication, letting go of grudges, and practicing forgiveness. Relationships are harmed when we harbor grudges, but they heal, flourish, and expand when we forgive.

Be present and show appreciation

Focus your whole attention on the people you're talking to. Be genuinely curious, pay close attention, and interact with the other person without any interruptions. Show your loved ones how much they mean to you by telling them how grateful you are for them. You should honor their achievements, recognize their contributions, and thank them for being there.

Using these methods, you may build and sustain connections that will enrich your life with love and companionship. Never forget that maintaining healthy relationships takes work, tolerance, and honesty. The benefits of love, friendship, and shared experiences can be felt at any stage of life, but especially as we age, so it's important to take the time to cultivate meaningful relationships.

Strategies to foster community involvement

Getting involved in your community is a great way to meet new people, make a positive impact, and feel more at home where you live. Methods to encourage participation in local affairs are as follows:

Volunteer

Volunteer in a way that makes sense for you and your beliefs. Seek out local groups or issues that you feel connected to and give your services to them. Participating in volunteer work is a great way to give back to the community, expand your social circle, and make new friends.

Join community groups

Join a club or organisation in your area and get involved. Groups like these can be anything from a reading club or sports team to a hobby society or a neighborhood watch. Participating in activities with people who share your interests opens the door to new friendships and experiences.

Attend community events

Take part in local gatherings such as fairs, festivals, conferences, and workshops. Meeting new people, learning about alternative points of view, and participating in group conversations and activities all help bring people together at these sorts of gatherings. Taking part in local gatherings is a great way to meet new people and establish ties within your neighborhood.

Support local businesses

Try to spend your money in places that are close to you. Support local businesses like bookstores, grocery stores, and restaurants to strengthen ties within the neighborhood. By patronizing locally owned establishments, you contribute to a healthy and prosperous neighborhood.

Participate in community service projects

Participate in volunteer efforts that help those in need or advance the community as a whole. This could include things like helping the environment, holding fundraisers, or cleaning up the neighborhood. Volunteering is a great way to meet new people and develop a sense of community because you'll be helping others while helping yourself.

Attend town hall meetings or community forums

Participate in community debates and learn more about local concerns by going to town hall meetings or forums. You can share your thoughts, participate in community decision-making, and meet people who share your interests and goals thanks to these channels.

Support community initiatives

Keep abreast of local causes and campaigns you may join. For causes that matter to you and your community, you may show your support by signing petitions, spreading the word on social media, and otherwise getting involved in advocacy activities. Contributing to community efforts shows that you care about the well-being of the area and inspires others to do the same.

Engage in intergenerational activities

It's important to actively seek out opportunities to engage in intergenerational activities. This could be accomplished through engagement in mentorship programs, service at youth centers, or attendance at gatherings for people of all ages. Participating in intergenerational activities helps people of all ages learn from one another and develops stronger bonds between generations.

These methods will help you become more involved in your neighborhood, make new friends, and improve the area. Community involvement has multiplicative effects, improving the lives of both the individual and the community at large. Participate actively in your community, and you'll see how it improves not only your life but the lives of those around you.

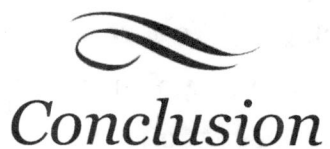

Conclusion

In this book, we've covered ground on the fundamentals of aging and holistic health. Let's review what we've covered thus far:

- We began by discussing what it means to be healthy and looking at the aging process from both a medical and psychological angle. We emphasized the need for a comprehensive view of aging that takes into account physical, mental, social, and spiritual health.

- We talked about the importance of getting the right mix of nutrients in your diet and why that's so important. We also understood how important water is to good health and longevity.

- We discussed what constitutes a "superfood," and how antioxidants affect the aging process. We included an exhaustive catalog of superfoods and the advantages they offer.

- We reviewed the importance of supplements and focused on the most crucial ones for healthy aging, such as vitamins, minerals, probiotics, omega-3 fatty acids, and collagen. We covered the benefits and drawbacks of using supplements and gave advice on how to choose the best ones.

- We identified healthy habits as a whole and highlighted their significance. We provided realistic strategies for a greener lifestyle, including swapping out hazardous cleaning supplies, eating more organic foods, and using less plastic. The effects of a healthy lifestyle on becoming older were examined.

- We discussed the multiple physiological and psychological advantages of maintaining an exercise routine. Cardiovascular activity, strength training, and alternative practices like yoga and Pilates were all covered. We recommended ways to make exercise a regular part of life.

- Mindfulness and meditation, cognitive exercises, and stress management are just some of the mental health care methods we covered, along with their relationship to aging. We underlined how a cheerful outlook might slow down the aging process.

- We discussed the importance of sleep to health and longevity, provided strategies to enhance the quality of sleep, and suggested solutions to common sleep problems. We emphasized that getting enough sleep is crucial to your health and should be a top priority.

- We acknowledged the role of social interaction in aging and researched methods of fostering community involvement and healthy relationships. We highlighted the significance of social interactions in fostering happiness and a healthy way of life as we age.

As we wrap up this book, we hope that it inspires you to take steps toward your own holistic health. Put into practice the newfound wisdom and understanding. Take care of your body, mind, and spirit by eating well, staying hydrated, and taking any necessary vitamins. Adopt a healthy lifestyle by eating right, exercising frequently, and cultivating your mind with techniques like meditation, cognitive retraining, and stress reduction. Spend enough time in bed each night and work on strengthening your relationships. Take part in civic life and make a positive impact on the lives of those around you.

Inspirations and closing thoughts

Never lose sight of the fact that growing older is its own beautiful adventure, ripe with chances to learn and experience more. Accept the inevitable aging changes and struggles, understanding that you have control over your own health and quality of life as you age. You can improve the quality of your life and age with dignity and vigor by giving equal importance to your mental, emotional, and physical well-being.

We hope this book will be a resource for you as you pursue holistic health and longevity. Put your faith in yourself and you will have a successful and exciting life. I wish you nothing but happiness, love, and plenty as you set off on your path today. Keep in mind that you can mature with dignity if you take care of yourself holistically and enjoy all that life has to offer.